# Cancer Battle – from a Patient's Perspective

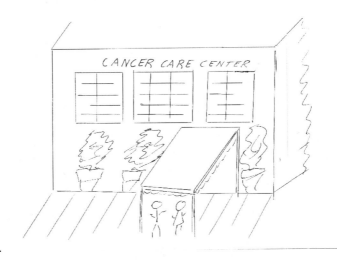

## Richard Larkin

## Reader Comments

"Wow. That was quite a journey for me as a reader. You really did a good job of explaining what you had experienced and in such a way which was scary, but positive with some humor as well.

Well done, you have done a good job and I'm sure it will help many people going through what you experienced or just beginning their journey."

L R. (UK)

# DEDICATION

This cancer guide was written for and is dedicated to all the medical professionals who are devoting their research, practice, and skills to helping reduce or eliminate cancer with its devastating effect on families and individuals throughout the world.

In addition, it is dedicated to my strong supporters where I work as a volunteer at the Mission Creek Correction Center for Women and I offer my thanks for all their prayers and good wishes as they work through far more difficult recovery programs than I have experienced as a cancer patient.

It is also dedicated to the individuals currently receiving cancer treatment, cancer survivors, and those who did not survive their battle with the disease. May they rest in peace.

# WHY DID THIS HAPPEN TO ME?

*According to the American Cancer Society Web site:*

*People with cancer often ask, "What did I do wrong?" or "Why me?" Doctors don't know for sure what causes cancer. When doctors can't give a cause, people may come up with their own ideas about why it happened. Most people wonder if they did something to cause the cancer.*

*If you're having these feelings, you're not alone. Thoughts and beliefs like this are common for people with cancer. Try not to blame yourself or focus on looking for ways you might have prevented cancer. Cancer is not your fault, and there's almost never a way to find out what caused it. Instead, focus on taking good care of yourself now.*

*Your American Cancer Society can tell you more about cancer and cancer treatment. Call 1-800-227-2345 anytime, day or night.*

# I was diagnosed with cancer – and it is scary

This writing is intended to share the experience of cancer treatment from a patient's perspective to help newly diagnosed cancer patients and medical providers improve their understanding of what goes through the mind of a patient as they work with their team of medical professionals trying to defeat their cancer.

# Table of Contents

# INTRODUCTION AND DIAGNOSIS

## Why I am writing this

Mentally and emotionally I was totally unprepared for my cancer journey, but as I began to experience several stages of treatment I realized most patients were probably in the same situation. I decided to write about cancer treatment from the eyes of a patient to share my observations and to help others understand a little more about what to expect as they fight their own battle. I cannot presume the reader will understand my "eyes" or perspective without some information about my medical history leading up to my cancer treatment.

## Brief Medical History

At the time of this writing I am 77 years old. Young to me, not necessarily to others. Doctor visits were never a high priority to me because I considered myself very healthy and felt I could work through most aches and pains without outside medical help. Other than 2 surgeries to repair some knee damage from a fall during a hike in the Northwest Cascade Mountains, my "normal" medical experience was to see a doctor about once or twice a year for prescription refills or occasional aches that did not clear up on their own.

## My journey through the cancer process

My journey began with an annual visit to my primary care physician for a renewal of my regular prescriptions. During the visit, I mentioned to her that I had been experiencing some bleeding with my bowel movements. I had occasionally had rectal bleeding over a few years and it always cleared up, so I never mentioned the incidents to her. In this case, she nicely but firmly pushed for a colonoscopy, something I had never agreed to before. On November 1, 2016 I had my first colonoscopy – and my life changed forever.

The doctor performing the procedure was a very kind individual who understood my anxiety level – not from any concern I had about cancer, but from a procedure that I considered invasive. When the procedure was over, and I was becoming clear headed he told me he had found a very concerning polyp (he might have said tumor) and I should meet an Oncologist as soon as possible. His nurse overheard the conversation and recommended seeing a doctor at St. Anthony Hospital in Gig Harbor, Washington.

# LEARNING WHAT TO EXPECT

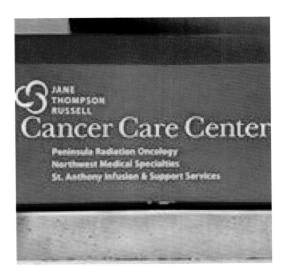

*Walking up to the Cancer Center brought back memories of arriving at Lockland AFB for Air Force basic training many years before – my initial thought was:*

*Uh oh, what have I just gotten myself into that I cannot back out of or change?*

As I walked toward the Cancer Center my wife was with me, so I was trying to be strong and keep my emotions to myself. When we opened the door to the reception area it hit me. I have visited many friends and relatives in hospitals over the years, but I had never paid any attention to the Cancer section. I began to realize I was not visiting, I was the patient.

I knew I was entering an area I was totally unfamiliar with and was about to start a journey I knew nothing about. I would not say I was fearful, but my anxiety level as we opened the door to the waiting area was many, many times higher than it was for the colonoscopy I had experienced a few days earlier.

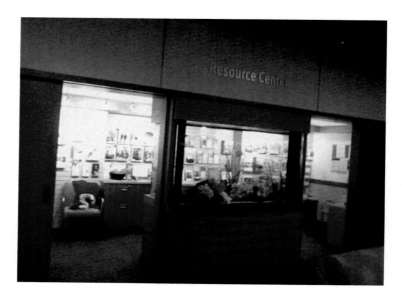

As we entered the waiting area, I was amazed. It was large, clean, nicely decorated with soothing colors, and all the furniture was comfortable and in good repair. It was designed to welcome and relax people who were functioning at a high stress level.

Taking it all in for the first time, I saw a large aquarium, tables with puzzles in work, a room full of helpful information for people to take home and read about various types of cancer and treatments, a free book exchange, sitting arrangements for people to wait with their friends and relatives without encroaching on their neighbors, and some of the best coffee I have ever enjoyed.

There were glassed in counters located around the room for specialty areas, or departments – Radiation, Hematology, Oncology, a Laboratory, a Cancer Navigator and others. The "departments" had names I did not recognize or understand, so I just went to the first counter and asked how to reach my scheduled appointment. The receptionist was very friendly, checked me in, and had us wait in the reception area.

*It is worth pointing out that as I have found my way through every one of the specialty areas of the Cancer Care Center, I have never had to wait more than ten minutes to meet the Doctor, Nurse, or other Practitioner for my scheduled appointment.*

*They are outstanding when it comes to respecting the patient's time – they also never make a patient feel rushed when they are with them.*

## Meeting the Doctor (the Oncologist)

Shortly after the receptionist checked me in (two days after my colonoscopy) I met the person who was to be my Oncologist with the Cancer Care Center, a part (separate wing) of a very large and somewhat overwhelming hospital.

I found the Oncologist to be a very warm, caring, knowledgeable, and reassuring cancer specialist who explained that I had been diagnosed with Malignant Neoplasm of the rectum and that it could be treated with radiation and chemotherapy. He told me I would be wearing a colostomy bag for the rest of my life.

WOW! I had no idea what all the information meant, in fact until I was talking to one I did not even know there was a medical specialist called an Oncologist.

*A doctor who has special training in diagnosing and treating cancer using chemotherapy, hormonal therapy, biological therapy, and targeted therapy.*

*A medical* **ONCOLOGIST** *often is the main health care provider for someone who has cancer – the team leader for the patient's cancer battle.*

He told me with my wife by my side, that it was not likely to be life threatening, but it would certainly change my lifestyle (I think he referred to it as changing my "quality of life").

He told us my cancer was advanced and we could not waste time starting the battle. The treatment he explained was going to start with 28 daily doses of radiation along with oral chemo therapy (pills) to be taken on the same days as the radiation. Due to Thanksgiving and the Christmas Holiday season, my radiation treatments went over a longer calendar time than a patient would normally spend. My radiation began on November 18, 2016 and finished on January 3, 2017.

## Orientation

After meeting with my Oncologist, my wife joined me for an orientation session which was a one-on-one session with a Cancer Center nurse. All I can say about the orientation is "overwhelming." The person explaining the radiation and chemotherapy process was like the other staff, very understanding and as informative as she could be.

From a patient's point of view, there was far too much information coming toward me at one time for me to grasp it. I still did not really understand what having cancer meant to an individual.

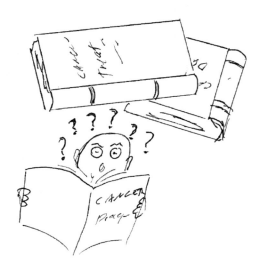

## Cancer Navigator

Following the orientation, we were introduced to a person known as the Cancer Navigator, a nurse with specialized training to help cancer patients throughout their treatment process.

The Navigator is available to help facilitate care and appointments, answer any questions related to individual needs, listen to concerns and help with referrals that may be necessary.

My first reaction was – it is nice to know she is here, but I'm quite capable of finding my way through the process. Boy was I wrong! The Cancer Navigator became a major player for me. She helped me when I did not even know I needed help – and was always available to share a smile and keep my spirits up. She will come up again in this writing to point out how she helped along the way.

My suggestion to any new cancer patient is:

get to know the Cancer Navigator – it will make your journey far more pleasant and you will always know you have an insider working with you.

# BEGINNING THE TREATMENT PROCESS

### Radiation therapy and oral chemo treatment

What I consider the first major battle in my fight with cancer was going through the combination of *radiation therapy* and *chemo treatment*. The radiation was a bit of an adventure, which I will explain beginning with the section "before radiation treatment."

## Chemo during radiation

The chemo (during this phase of the cancer battle) was very important to the doctors, but from my perspective it was not difficult. The chemo was in the form of pills taken each day while I went to the radiation machine. The pills had a bad taste and I think they were more potent than I understood at the time since they could only be dispensed by the Cancer Care unit of the hospital. They could not be purchased at a regular pharmacy.

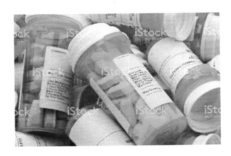

*Cancer Navigator help* – this was the first time I went to the Cancer Navigator to help me understand what I was doing. The instructions on the chemo pill bottles might have been clear for medical people, but as I read the dosage instructions and had my wife read them too, we did not agree on how many pills I was supposed to take each day.

I showed the Cancer Navigator the bottles and *she broke the code*. She was able to understand how many pills the Oncologist and Pharmacist said I should take each day – so off I went with the oral chemo portion of my treatment under control.

_Side effects_

I had been warned about all kinds of potential side effects from the pills, but luckily in my experience, I had almost no side effects from the chemo pills. I was not getting nauseated which I guess had been expected because they gave me three types of pills to minimize the effect. I never took any of the anti-nausea pills. I was a little dizzy at times, but it was pretty mild and I seemed to be able to control it by wandering (carefully) in the yard – focusing on plants instead of myself.

I suppose if there was an overriding side effect throughout my cancer battle it would be fatigue and some mental confusion which falls under the medical term: chemo brain.

_Example of chemo brain:_

_I said to my wife one day "let's go out to the backyard and soak up some Sun." She agreed and went to the backyard, I went to the front deck and wondered where she was. Chemo brain does not stop a person from functioning, and if a person can learn to laugh at it, it is not anything to fear._

They assured me that all the side effects would wear off over time when the cancer battle is concluded, but it could go on for weeks, months, or more.

Side effects from <u>radiation</u> – a different story and not much fun. They will be described as I discuss the radiation treatment process.

I should probably admit to another side effect that is usually not included in the "list" they provide to help a patient cope with the cancer battle. This side effect they do not seem to discuss would be tears. Yes, tears – feeling a bit sorry for myself.

I was brought up in a generation like many before mine, where men did not show many emotions. We were supposed to be strong and comfort women when they felt bad, but remain strong and not let others know if we were feeling down. It did not work too well this time. Though I managed to keep most of my "emotions" to myself around others while they said "you look good," most people did not seem to understand that my inner self was feeling pretty bad and I was feeling sorry for myself.

As my treatment went on I continued to work on my emotional side. I realized I was entering a new lifestyle, not ending a life, so I needed to adapt. I found it helped a lot to wander in the yard with nature and return my focus toward trying to help other people who had more problems than I did. My "poor me" attitude (though still with me a bit) began to mellow.

## Before Radiation treatment

Before starting the radiation sessions, I had a Magnetic Resonance Imaging (MRI) and a Computed Tomography (CT) scan. They sound like a big deal, but to a patient they are actually quite relaxing. In both cases I just laid on a moving table and let my mind wander to places unknown while I was moved back and forth through a big round donut hole. I had to remain as still as possible so my only problem was trying not to fall asleep during the procedure.

The "action" as I think of the cancer battle began after the MRI and CT were completed. I met the next Doctor in my new world, referred by title as a Radiation Oncologist. Before I met him, he had thoroughly reviewed my medical records and the MRI, CT scan images. Like the Oncologist he was a very kind, caring, and knowledgeable Doctor who gave me every reason to completely trust him through his amazing knowledge of my personal cancer situation, his positive body language, and his easy to understand explanation of what to expect during the radiation sessions.

He went over my situation in detail and helped me know what to expect with each visit, the potential side effects, and what I might feel physically during the process. It was a very open discussion and he responded to all questions or concerns I had or my wife had at the time.

My wife was with me during doctor to review test results and as they explained a new procedure (e.g. radiation, surgery, etc.) when it was about to begin so we could compare what we heard as we both tried to understand each phase of the cancer battle. She did not accompany me when I went for tests or routine procedures.

In addition to daily radiation treatments, the Radiation Oncologist scheduled one-on-one weekly visits so he could hear in detail how I was doing and when necessary, provide advice and/or prescriptions to offset some of the burning sensations I would be experiencing.

## PET Scan

Due to my type of cancer, its stage of development and its location, he suggested having a PET Scan before he went into what he referred to as a "very labor intensive" programming of the radiation equipment.

> *Positron Emission Tomography (PET) is an imaging device that allows a doctor to check for diseases in a person's body. It uses a special dye with radioactive tracers injected into a vein in the arm. The body's organs and tissues absorb the tracer. When highlighted under a PET scanner, the tracers help a doctor understand how well all organs and tissues are working. The PET scan can measure blood flow, oxygen use, glucose metabolism (how the body uses sugar), and much more.*

*When a PET Scan is used to detect cancer, it allows the doctor to see how the cancer metabolizes and whether it has spread or metastasized to new areas. Used after treatment, PET can also show how a tumor is responding to chemotherapy.*

So – off I went to have a PET Scan. What a relaxing experience it turned out to be. As usual, I started by meeting a nice receptionist who gave me a lot of paperwork to fill out.

Every step along the way required the same paperwork to be filled out related to my medical history, insurance, etc. yet, when I met with practitioners they all had a computer screen in front of them showing my complete medical history.

The question in my mind is:

If each hospital department and Doctor's office has all of my medical information in their interconnected computer system, why do I have to fill out the same paperwork for each receptionist? Just a question. I never brought it up because I wanted to stay on their good side (I wanted them to like me) and I know they were just doing their job.

## PET Scan Procedure

My first step of having the PET Scan was to go into a private little room and remove my street clothes, put on a hospital gown, and lay down on a very comfortable bed. When the nurse came back, she injected the radioactive dye into my arm (no pain, not really any feeling to it) and covered me with a heated blanket. She dimmed the lighting in the room and I think I might even remember her turning on soft music. It was a totally relaxing experience while I rested and we waited for the dye to work its way through my body.

When the time was right (probably about an hour, maybe far less – I really did not know), I was moved to the PET Scan machine.

Like the MRI and CT imaging I had earlier, the PET Scan was totally painless and relaxing for me. It was a little boring because my function was to simply stay still on a moving table while it slid back and forth through a big round hole.

From the technician's part of the experience, I imagine it required more hands-on activity. I simply laid on my sliding table, tried again not to fall asleep while I waited for them to tell me I was finished and could go home.

# EXPERIENCING RADIATION TREATMENT

## Planning radiation treatment

Now comes the real action – the tests were finished, the Radiation Oncologist had reviewed them and completed programming the radiation machine – I was about to start 28 sessions of radiation treatment.
During the live radiation treatment, a patient must try to remain totally motionless in the area where they are shooting the machine rays (or whatever they might call them).

To be sure a patient remains motionless:

> They place 3 small tattoos (about the size of a pencil point) near the area where the radiation will be entering the patient's body. (I think) they are used to align laser beams with each session so the radiation machine will point to exactly the same place every time it is used.

They make a brace for each individual. Depending upon the cancer target area (location of the tumor), they might use a face mask, headrest, plaster cast, or some other similar device. My brace was easy for me. They created two molded braces so I could put my legs in them to keep from moving my lower abdomen – the target area for colorectal cancer.

## _Simulating radiation treatment_

Before the live radiation began, they had me take part in a simulation so I would know my role and what was expected of me during each session. It was about the same as actors do before their first stage play when they have a dress rehearsal – they go through the entire play without a paying audience.

Working with the radiation professionals who were with me for each session, they showed me how to prepare for the radiation, how to get on the table next to what I refer to as a monster robot and place my legs against my braces, and how to lay while the machine was running.

A typical radiation machine is shown in this picture:

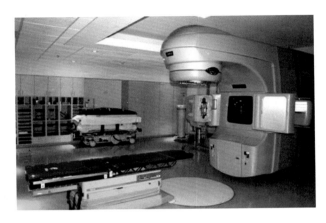

## *Live radiation treatments*

The treatment is technically (I think) called *External-beam radiation therapy*. While I laid motionless on the table, the monster robot moved over me and made a series of noises as it gradually circled my lower abdomen for 15 minutes.
I was scheduled for 28 radiation sessions 5 times a week (Monday through Friday). My sessions which started on November 18 would have ended without holidays on December 27. Since my treatments overlapped with the Thanksgiving, Christmas, and New Year holidays, my last session was January 3.

The early sessions were fine. No pain, no side effects, no problem that had me very concerned. I was even thinking "if this is all there is to fighting cancer, no big deal. I can handle it." Boy did I have a lot to learn – very quickly.

By about the third week, I began feeling what I had been warned might be like a Sunburn in areas where we don't usually get a Sunburn. How true! The pain (I think from hitting each tattoo with a laser with each session) was beginning to grow. In addition, my entire lower abdomen was getting very raw on the surface and apparently on the inside from the radiation.

The Doctor was very understanding and prescribed creams to help minimize the pain. When medical professionals asked about my pain level on a scale from 1 to 10 with 10 being high, I always said mine was 13. (I talked with another patient going through the same treatment in the same area who rated the pain level at 50). *The pain does pass and is eventually forgotten.*

I began to look forward to weekends and holiday's so I could have a short break between sessions and the pain would drop a little, though I also knew what to expect when I returned Monday and was back on the radiation table.

As other phases of my cancer battle continued, I would often see the Radiation Technician in the waiting area getting ready to escort a person into the Radiation Room. I would always stop and say a brief hello to him – and thank him for doing his part in my battle. It brought a smile from him and I think it helped him know he was a positive part of helping people survive.

# LITTLE REWARDS

As the radiation therapy went on and my pain level increased, I decided I needed some target or goal to shoot for to get me through each session. I found it in the form of a paper coffee cup. I set a goal of trying to be fully cooperative and present a positive attitude throughout each procedure. When I completed the "procedure" I gave myself a *little reward* – an excellent cup of coffee to enjoy on my way home.

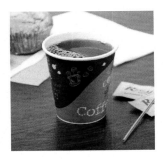

The coffee came from a counter in the Cancer Center waiting room with some of the best tasting fresh coffee I have ever enjoyed. It was free, it was always fresh, and it became a special place for me.

*The coffee is brewed and taken care of by the Radiation Oncology Department Receptionist, one if the nicest people on our planet – so if you ever enjoy some of her coffee, please stop by and let her know how much you appreciate it.*

I began to notice routines in the waiting area of the Cancer Center. Different days brought different groups of people and activities. Some days a person would be playing the harp or teaching a group of people how to play a harp. Sometimes it would be a group of cancer patients sitting in a circle quietly talking and knitting.

Sometimes it was a visit by Griffin.

# Say hello to Griffin

Tuesday usually brought a visit from a therapy dog named Griffin.

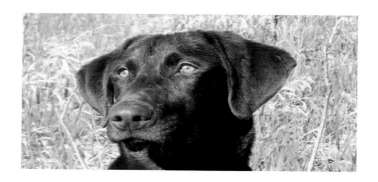

Griffin went to each patient and let them pet and talk with him. There was a noticeable relaxation in the patient's body language when the dog was with them.

Note: I was referring to Griffin as a *service dog* until his handler told me he was *a therapy dog* – different from a service dog.

A service dog is specialized, or trained to perform a specific task such as directing a blind person, letting a person know if the telephone is ringing, watching for potential falls, etc.
A therapy dog is more generalized. Like our buddy Griffin, they help several people, not just the person they are assigned to. For example, Griffin visits patients in all areas in the hospital (probably not during surgery) whether they are in a bed, sitting in a chair, or standing nearby.

I could see that the individuals looked forward to their routine activities and within a few weeks, I was taking part in some of the activities– not knitting, but meeting people and listening to their stories.

I found that every person was fighting their own battle, but they were all trying to keep a sense of humor, share stories about their lives, and keep other people around them smiling.

*I found it interesting that adults fighting cancer and knowing the result if they lose the battle tend to talk about their adult life far more than their youth or raising a family. They are not caught up in a "poor me" attitude, but they tend to enjoy sharing later accomplishments.*

## Learning about life

After a few radiation sessions I realized I was seeing the same people leaving just before I went into my treatment. Patient scheduling brought us together at the same time.

When I came out from the radiation the same man was always waiting to enter and we began to chat a bit while we crossed paths. I was building a relationship with him and when we learned our pre-retirement (and pre-cancer) lives were very similar, we discussed meeting to share stories after our cancer battles were concluded.

It did not work out. His cancer spread and he passed away just as we were getting to know each other. He was the first person I met in the Cancer unit that died while I was experiencing my battle. I'm sorry to say he was not the last. He was an important element in my *learning about life* and beginning to realize cancer is not a game.

# PREPARING FOR THE FIRST SURGERY

## Rest and prepare for surgery

Ah! Time to relax and recuperate from the radiation therapy. The next step in my battle was to be surgery –it did not sound like fun, but at least I had a recovery period of a few weeks to not think much about it. Apparently, the timing of surgery after radiation treatment is critical. The body needs to be ready to take new cutting and pasting by a surgeon before scar tissue resulting from radiation therapy develops too much to work with. What it meant to me was I had a few weeks to enjoy and not visit the Cancer Unit.

> *Colorectal surgery*
> The planned surgery was to remove my rectum and the cancer tumor which was too close to the opening to save the rectum. They were also adding a large intestine outlet referred to as a "colostomy" to my front near my stomach. The surgery will be discussed in some detail a little later in this writing. *(I was finding out more about what the Oncologist meant during our first meeting when he said I was going to have a "life changing" experience).*

At this time in my cancer battle, my job was to relax. The radiation had done a lot to stir up the inner and outer portions of my lower abdomen and they told me I needed a few weeks for my body to settle down before I have surgery.

My own thinking at the time of this writing was I had been through over seven months of radiation and taking powerful pills. I was looking forward to a lot more than a few weeks for my "body to settle down."

## The Surgeon

As my rest period began (estimated to be about six weeks), I went with my wife to meet the surgeon. Like all the other medical professionals I had met so far, she was very nice, very knowledgeable about the surgery, my medical history, and our anxiety level. She set the tone of our first (and all follow-on meetings) by shaking hands and saying hello, I am Linda. She did not enter with an air of superiority, but instead she met us with body language that said we were the important people in the room and we had her full attention.

She explained what to expect with the surgery and what life would be like after the surgery. She did it very well, but like every other phase of my battle, we did not understand all of the information and we both went away with slightly different opinions of what Linda had told us. Nevertheless, we were comfortable and knew we would learn more before the actual surgery.

So – the rest period. I actually had only two weeks before I met again for a status meeting with my primary Oncologist, then two more weeks before a follow-up discussion with the surgeon. These meetings were fine with me since I was not involved in any actual "procedures" at the time – I was just resting and spending days as I had before beginning the radiation therapy.

The rest really helped. Over time the pain from radiation and lasers was leaving and I was really feeling good. It felt great, but my life was heading for another modification.

The **Urologist**

While the Radiation Oncologist was reviewing the results of my PET Scan, he saw a small dot on a kidney. This had been studied by a Urologist nearly 15 years earlier and ended up to be nothing to get excited about.

> A few years earlier we moved to a new home so the original Urologist was a long way from the Cancer Center where my battle was being conducted.

Due to my new cancer situation, the Radiation Oncologist suggested having a nearby Urologist check my kidney with Ultrasound while I was in the hospital to see if anything had changed from earlier medical images and whether it was becoming an area of concern. The Radiation Oncologist recommended a Urologist to me and I went to meet him – big mistake!!!

I'm trying to keep names out of this writing and focus on neutrality from the eyes of a patient, but I would suggest to any reader (potential patient) if you are considering going to a Urologist about two traffic circles from St. Anthony Hospital, do some research first.

When I went to my appointment (during my pre-surgery rest period) with the Urologist, I had just completed my 28 radiation treatments. My "male parts" were still very painful and I was a long way from feeling normal. I went to him thinking we would discuss having an ultrasound check of my kidney in the hospital. He was not planning on any "discussion." He was already to poke a camera into my bladder.

I told the Urologist my bladder was fine and I was in far too much pain to let him poke me with a camera. I guess it would be accurate to say our conversation did not go well and we did not appear to be heading toward a comfortable doctor/patient relationship.

We concluded the appointment with no camera activity and I ended up scheduling another appointment with him, though with hindsight I don't know why I agreed to another appointment.

My second appointment with the Urologist was the day before my scheduled surgery. His idea was to check my bladder before surgery so if anything went poorly during the surgery he would know what had changed. I agreed and he went in to my bladder with his camera.

Ouch! I have had a camera inserted there before, but never as painfully as his camera. He did not numb anything in advance, which other Urologists had done, and he seemed to be much slower with his procedure when compared to previous experiences. I don't think he liked me and he was taking it out on me – can't say for sure, but it is my patient perspective.

When he finished, he told me I needed bladder surgery to stop frequent urination and minimize the urge to go. I did not even bother to tell him I don't experience those symptoms and all of the scans other doctors had reviewed so far did not show any bladder problem.

He scheduled a pre-surgery appointment – good luck on seeing me again. I agreed to the scheduling so I could get out of his office, then by telephone a few days later I cancelled it.

So, as I said earlier "…if you are considering going to a Urologist about two traffic circles from St. Anthony Hospital, do some research first" and insist on a second opinion.

I probably should say at this point, my cancer battle covered nearly a year of active medical procedures. The only negative and non-professional medical person I was involved with was the Urologist. Every other person on the Cancer Center and Hospital from the Doctors to and including the janitors were totally professional, caring, and a pleasure to work with.

Note: Multiple tests and procedures after surgery in the Intensive Care Unit verified the dot on my kidney was not a concern – no matter what the Urologist said. In fact, he never looked at or checked the kidney – the reason I went to see him in the first place.

# INTRODUCING THE COLOSTOMY BAG

## What is a Colostomy?

Sometimes, for medical reasons, part of the large bowel (colon and rectum) has to be removed or bypassed. This means that bowel movements can no longer be passed out of the body through the anus in the usual way. Therefore an operation is performed to create a new opening on the front of the abdomen.

The colon is brought out through the skin to form a colostomy. This new outlet is pink and moist like the inside of the mouth and is called a stoma. A removable plastic bag is attached to the skin around the stoma. If you need more information about the Colostomy bag, there is a lot on the Internet and in free booklets in Cancer Care Resource rooms and on the Internet.

*It sounds kind of unpleasant but over time it is OK – and other people do not see the bag.*

## Colostomy nurse

The location of the colostomy bag is determined by a specialist, a Colostomy Nurse. We went to meet her to learn more about the bag I would be wearing for the rest of my life – ugh.

She did an excellent job of explaining what I was getting into and how my life would be changing. She also assured me that I was not alone – there are thousands of people who wear the same kind of bag that I would be wearing, but in my mind I was thinking *"I appreciate having you tell me how others are doing with their bags, but in my spoiled frame of mind, this time it is about me, not another person."*

When she was finished with her explanations and she had answered all of our questions we had at the time, she concluded the session by using a black felt marker to draw a big dot (about 2 inch diameter) on my stomach. I was told to not wash it off because it was the location for the surgeon to place my bag. Ouch – reality keeps getting closer.


# THE FIRST SURGERY

## Lab tests – and hospital layout

A few days before the scheduled surgery, I was told to go to the lab test area and give blood to help the professionals prepare for my operation. Sounds easy, but it was quite confusing.

I went directly to the lab in the Cancer Unit near my Oncologist, the Radiation Therapy area, and other Cancer related sections. Wrong choice – I was informed that I was in the Cancer Lab, but my surgery was in a different (connected) building in the Hospital, therefore I had to go to the Hospital Lab. It worked out – long walk, but good exercise.

I think all hospitals have confusing layouts. It does not seem to be because of their initial design, but instead it is due to expansion over a long period of time. They build, they connect, and they use department labels that non-medical people don't always understand. With the right attitude, we can survive the confusion of hospitals by laughing at how silly we look as we keep ending up in odd locations a long way from where we are supposed to be going for our scheduled appointment.

After finding the right lab, I gave my blood and went home.

Suggestion – If I had taken my own advice and stopped by the Cancer Navigator before wandering all around the hospital looking for their lab, it would have saved time and been a little more efficient – so, once again: remember the Cancer Navigator, your helpful resource.

## Check-in

Now it was getting scary. I started this writing by saying as I entered the Cancer Care Center for the first time: *"Uh oh, what have I just gotten myself into that I cannot back out of or change?"* That was nothing compared to my anxiety level as I was checking into the surgical unit. Again, I was trying to appear strong for my wife who was with me, but inside I was as weak as a newborn baby and I wanted to run away from all of it.

The check-in process went smoothly and we were sent to a surgical waiting area a few floors away. The receptionist took my paperwork and showed us where to sit until they called us. This might have been a little calming if I had not looked at a wall with pictures of a lot of surgeons I assumed were like a Board of "Bosses." The alarming part was the picture right in the middle looking back at me was the Urologist who wanted to perform an unneeded bladder surgery on me. My anxiety rose when I saw him and thought the Hospital must like him – wow, do the even know about his "bedside manner."

## Pre-Operation

With very little wait time, we were ushered into an area I will refer to as the pre-operation unit where each person about to have surgery changes into a surgical gown, lays on a rolling bed, and they begin whatever preparation is necessary before entering the actual operating room.

While waiting in the pre-operation unit, I received a visit by the surgeon with some calming words to let me relax a little. Then I was visited by the Anesthesiologist to discuss his role in the surgery – keep me alive and under his chemically induced control (I think he used better medical terminology). I told him I did not want to hear or see anything and he assured me I would not be aware of anything during the surgery.

## The surgery

My surgery was scheduled to start at 5:15 AM and was expected to last about 5 hours.

It did not work out that way – I'm not sure why it went longer, but I was told the surgery went a few hours longer than expected – they told me I was suspended upside down for several hours.

I'm not sure what suspended up-side-down means, but I never wanted to ask for details.

I was scheduled to have surgery on February 9 and "probably" go home February 15 – it did not happen that way. I had some problems during recovery which I will explain under the heading *"heading for pneumonia."*

When they rolled me into the Operating room it was surprisingly bright, large, and full of complicated looking equipment. Several people in the room introduced themselves to me and told me what they would be doing.

The Anesthesiologist said he was going to start his drugs, I said "OK" – and that was the last thing I remembered until I was in the Post-Surgery area and someone was saying "wake up, it is time to wake up." **Then my battle with cancer took on a whole new look – and not in a good way.**

## Recovery after surgery

I remember very little about being moved into the hospital recovery area (not sure I have the right name – but it is where people go for a few days until they are ready to go home).
I don't remember any of the "recovery" process, but I do know I had visitors. I don't remember the visits, but I could tell by cards, magazines, etc. who had been by to see me – though I did not read any of them until I checked out of the hospital and was home. (My vision was too fuzzy from medications to read).

My wife told me she visited every day and, after she mentioned it I do vaguely remember playing a short dice game with her. I don't remember the actual game, but there is a hazy memory of our shaking dice and keeping a score pad.

I was told I was doing alright in the recovery process over a few days, though I was also told (I don't remember) I was very reluctant to get up and walk due to my pain. I have since learned how important it is to walk following surgery, even with pain – to get the body moving again and minimize congestion.

About the third day following surgery (I am just guessing at the time since I don't remember very much of the experience) my wife said she came to visit and found my bed empty and the room I was in cleaned of all of my personal things.

A message I'm writing to the hospital staff – this was bad. After nearly 50 years of marriage and having watched other people we have known die in a hospital, the empty room with no indication of where I had gone was pretty shocking to her and could have caused some problems (fainting, etc.).

A nurse saw her and told her the hospital had called her cell phone to let her know I had been moved to Intensive Care. The problem is, we do not touch our cell phones when we drive, so she did not answer the call.

Suggestion: If a hospital moves a patient, why not place a note on the room door telling where to find the patient? At least keep the note on the door until a new patient is moved into the room.

# ASPIRATION PNEUMONIA

ASPIRATION PNEUMONIA is an infection that inflames the air sacs in one or both lungs. The air sacs may fill with fluid or pus (purulent material), causing cough with phlegm or pus, fever, chills, and difficulty breathing.

## Heading for pneumonia

This segment will explain some major problems I had as a result of the surgery – not the fault of any member of the surgical team, just bad luck on my part.

The details I'm about to describe are based upon discussions with my wife, doctors, nurses, and others involved with the surgery because I was mentally not aware of any of these events and I have no memory of them.

Apparently while I was in the recovery process, I began vomiting (sorry, I don't know a nice way to say it) and managed to get some bacteria into my lungs which, as near as I can understand is a cause of aspiration pneumonia – so off I went to the Intensive Care Unit.

## *Where did my brain go?*

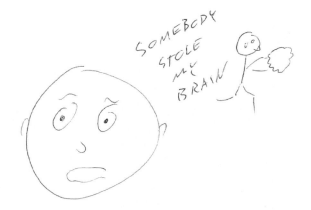

When I was heading for the Intensive Care Unit due to pneumonia, I was (in layman's terms) nuts. My brain was not under my control anymore.

I don't remember much of the experience, but I do remember being wheeled through the hospital shouting at people, telling them it was not a real hospital, and who knows what else. In other words, I was out of my mind and totally different from my regular self. I have no idea where the outburst was coming from or how long it lasted since I was in what I'd call a total mental fog.

**Advice for a person about to have surgery:** Don't read a mystery book or watch a -movie about a murder in a hospital a few days before checking in for your surgery. I did, and I think it might have influenced my thought processes.

It might be the reason airlines do not seem to show in-flight movies about airplanes crashing or being hijacked – not a good idea to for stressed out passengers to watch when they are 35,000 feet above ground in a sealed aluminum tube.

I think they gave me something to quiet me when I reached the Intensive Care Unit because the next time I remember talking with anyone, I was back to being a positive person and I had several intravenous (IV) tubes, pumping machines, and drains connected to me.

In my "normal" life, I'm as opposite from this episode as a person can get. I have spent decades studying Human Relations and teaching college students how to get along with other people.

In my life as a retiree I spend several hours a month donating my time to working one-on-one with inmates in the local Women's Correction Center to create business plans to help them develop self-esteem and see a positive future when they are released.

All I can say is somebody else had control of my brain – because it certainly was not my style.

## Intensive Care Unit (ICU)

Once again, I don't really know how long I was in the ICU, but it was long enough to get to know some of the nurses and hospital staff as they rotated through their shifts. I learned that there seem to be two types of nurse. They are all very well trained and excellent in their understanding of following a Doctor's orders and caring for each patient. They do differ, however, in their "bedside manner."

One type (my favorite) is not only very good about following the procedures (giving medicine at the right time, checking vital signs, etc.), but they appear to take a sincere interest in the patient. They listen to patient stories and as time goes on, they share some of their own experiences raising kids, hiking in the local area, etc. They are friendly, efficient, and I believe paying a lot of attention to a patient's progress while they are sharing stories.

The other type (my least favorite) is also very good about following procedures, but they go by the book. They do what they are told, they administer drugs with no idle chatter, and they seem to be totally caught up in doing things the way they were taught to, not taking into account that each patient is a unique individual with a high stress level and needs to maintain human to human contact.

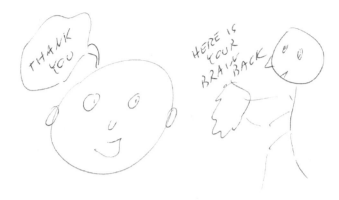

While my brain was returning to my control and still pretty fuzzy, I began to see some nurses with four eyes instead of two.  I never asked them about their eyes and as my head began to clear  I decided to keep that little secret to myself or I might be transferred to a mental institution.  Hopefully by now if I see the same people again, they will have only two eyes each.

As near as I can tell (again by hearing from other people), I was in Intensive Care for about a week.
Like the surgical recovery staff, they wanted me to get up and walk to help regain my strength and mobility.

It was very hard to do because the Intensive Care Unit has far more devices connected to patients than other areas I was in. About all I could do (with assistance) and a lot of pain was to stand, move to a chair, sit, then after a bit of time move back to the bed (a total "walk" of about 4 feet).

Eventually my brain seemed to be returning to normal. When I realized I had been suspended upside down during surgery it occurred to me that my pain might be from having my back bent awkwardly for a few hours – so I tried an experiment. When they helped me get out of the bed, I tried to straighten my back by reaching up with just one hand to a bar, pull straight up, and stand. It gave me one major jolt of pain, but I assumed that was my back trying to straighten out. Following the "jolt" the pain left and it felt alright to stand. With no pain, I felt like walking (using a walker) – and off I went with a nurse by my side.

After a day of walking further and further down the hall, the nurse asked me where I was going. When I said I had no pain and I enjoyed walking, he told me I had gone about 50 feet beyond my room. I just told him I was going home and would meet him in the parking lot. Not an acceptable plan with only my fancy hospital gown on.

## General comments about the Intensive Care Unit (ICU):

The hospital has a Doctor assigned to the ICU with responsibility for each patient's care. He is an extremely knowledgeable individual with a great bedside manner. He works directly with the surgeon and Oncologist but uses his own specialized training to treat the patient – in my case to fight the pneumonia.

In a very nice (not scary) way, when I was over pneumonia and heading back to the post-surgery recovery unit, he stopped by for a chat and he told me he was not sure I was going to survive when he first saw me. I'm certainly glad his medical training worked out – even though other than IV nourishment the only thing I was permitted to take by mouth during my ICU experience was shaved ice – kind of dull and no flavor.

## Return to post-surgery recovery

After I began walking in the ICU hallway, I was moved back to the post-surgery area and with a couple of days showing them how well I could move around I was cleared to go home. The only thing pacing my leaving the hospital was a required visit by the Colostomy Nurse to give me a little more training on how to work with my bag until they could get a visiting nurse to come to our home.

Interesting to note:

When my wife signed the discharge paperwork as my driver and at-home caregiver, *she had to sign a note saying she would not let me (the discharged patient) search the Internet* or look at any on-line sales sites for 24 hours.

I'm guessing they have had some fuzzy headed patients make interesting purchases when they went home.

## Spiritual Advisor

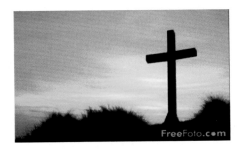

I was ready to go home and very anxious to get my final briefing from the Colostomy Nurse when a very nicely groomed lady came by to see me. She was wearing casual (not hospital) clothes, had nicely trimmed hair, and was probably around 60 years old. She looked like what I expected the nurse to look like so when she entered my room I said "boy am I glad to see you."

Right away I went into a series of questions about the bag on my stomach and she looked kind of confused. I looked at her hospital 1. D. badge and realized it said something about spiritual support and she had a bible in her hand. She was not the nurse I was waiting for, she was a spiritual advisor offering help to patients.

When I explained who I thought she was, we both laughed and had a nice conversation. On the way out she asked if I would like to have her say a prayer for me and I replied "oh boy you bet."

## Colostomy Nurse

The nurse did arrive and provided some very helpful training on how to change my bag which offset some of the fear of going home and having to take care of myself – it was kind of like taking home a newborn baby. All of a sudden you are on your own (as parents) and have to learn a lot of baby maintenance and training that is not shared in books.

I realized I still had more learning to do. I had to learn to handle living with my rectum removed and wearing a colostomy bag on my stomach for the rest of my life. Not much fun, but I was assured thousands of other people had been through it and there were a lot of caring professionals willing to help me along the way.

Since my release from the hospital, I've had my share of Colostomy bag bursting, leaking, etc. experiences. I (we) survived them as I have continued to learn how often to check it and change it. It is not much fun, but over time it is getting easier and easier to put up with.

If you are about to be introduced to a Colostomy bag, don't be afraid of it. I just think back on helping raise our children. A diaper change is never fun, but when it is finished everything is alright again and the child is happy.

## Home at last

My wife drove me home from the hospital – and even though I was a little dazed and very weak from spending so much time in a hospital bed with chemicals being fed into me, it was a great feeling to see our house, our yard, and a lot of familiar, comforting scenery.

The first thing I did when I entered our house was to head upstairs to our master bathroom to shave. That was a challenge. There are 14 steps to our second floor and each step felt like I was climbing a steep mountain trail. I made it to the top, shaved, and headed back down where I collapsed comfortably in an easy chair.

Good idea sort of – but not quite. The chair is very nice to sit in, but I had not realized until I became so weak that living room furniture tends to be quite low to the floor and as a result, very hard to get out of with weak muscles (my muscles had atrophied – become weak – from going so long with very little use).

I will end the discussion of my surgery and hospital stay in this writing by saying:

"I still had more learning to do and I was assured there were a lot of caring professionals willing to help me along the way."

# VISITING NURSE AND PHYSICAL THERAPIST

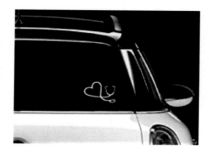

When people at the hospital told me "...there were a lot of caring professionals to help me along the way..." they were certainly correct. The "caring professionals" came in the form of a Home Physical Therapist, a Visiting Nurse and a volunteer handyman with Bluebills.

<u>Physical Therapist</u>

The first person to visit our home (within one day of checking out of the hospital) was a Physical Therapist. He had me walk, climb our stairway, and do various movements to see what he could do to help me take care of myself at home. He found that laying in a hospital bed had taken quite a toll on my muscle strength, so he showed me how to do some simple exercises to regain my strength and endurance.

Before he left, he set a visitation schedule for a different Physical Therapist to come by and help me with the exercises. Also, to keep me honest – without their regular visit it is very easy to put off doing the exercises on a regular basis.

In addition to scheduling regular visits by a Physical Therapist, he contacted Bluebills, an organization of retired Boeing workers who help people by donating their time to build wheel chair ramps, hand rails, and other fixtures around the house to improve safe mobility for recovering patients and elderly citizens.

Bluebills – Volunteer services for disabled

In my case, the Physical Therapist was concerned when he watched me try to get out of my chair, so he contacted Bluebills. The next day, a volunteer carpenter arrived and placed wooden risers under the chair I was using so I would not have to strain my knees getting into and out of the chair.

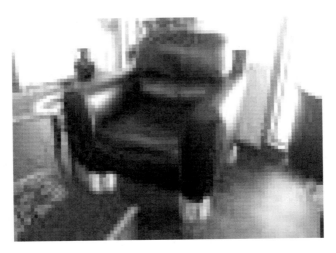

The risers will be returned to Bluebills when I am fully recovered and do not need them anymore.

## Visiting Nurse

Like the Bluebill carpenter, two days after checking out of the hospital, a vising nurse came to visit. She was great! She came by twice a week for several weeks and helped me understand and work with my Colostomy bag, she checked and replaced the silver dressing on my wound which I will be referring to soon under the heading "Wound Doctor."

The visiting nurse was my "rock" – my in-house medical professional who was available to answer questions, provide guidance, and help me through the transition from total hospital care to caring for myself.

It is an odd relationship with a visiting nurse and a physical therapist. We laughed together, shared experiences together, and built a trusting bond during the healing process. Eventually when it is time for them to go on to help others, the constant contact fades away. They leave behind a feeling of loss and questions about whether I can take care of myself, but they know when it is time – and their departure is for the good of all involved. It is like sending a new bird out of the nest – they (the bird and myself a patient) need to be on their own so they can survive and grow.

# CANCER TREATMENT AFTER FIRST SURGERY

## Next phase of Cancer Treatment

Very soon after I was released from the hospital we met with the Oncologist to learn how I was doing after radiation therapy and surgery:

- The radiation had killed the cancer near my rectum as well as some nearby lymph nodes.

  Definition: Lymph node (source: WWW.Cancer.gov/cancer terms)

  A small bean-shaped structure that is part of the body's immune system. Lymph nodes filter substances that travel through the lymphatic fluid, and they contain white blood cells that help the body fight infection and disease.

  There are hundreds of lymph nodes found throughout the body, Clusters of lymph nodes are found in the neck, axilla (underarm), chest, abdomen, and groin

- They were fairly certain, but not positive that there were no other lymph nodes with cancer floating around my body.

- If there were cancerous lymph nodes remaining, they could bump into lungs, the liver, or some other critical area and start spreading more aggressive cancer.

Because of the uncertainty related to possible cancerous lymph nodes still in my body, he recommended another phase of cancer treatment using IV chemotherapy. He said my chance of getting all the cancer out of my body by using the IV procedure was 90%. If I did not go for the IV procedure he estimated a 55% chance of survival. I chose to go for the IV treatment and entered a new phase of my journey.

### Intravenous chemotherapy (IV)

Treatment in which anticancer drugs are given through a needle or tube inserted into a vein. The anticancer drugs travel through the blood to kill cancer cells in the body.

### IV Port – another surgery

Having anticancer drugs (chemo) by IV is a simple, but repetitive process. It requires several weeks of having blood tests and sitting for hours at a time with bags "dripping" cancer fighting fluids (referred to by most of us as "chemo" into the bloodstream. Some people have their IV done through injections into veins in their arms. I chose to have a port installed to avoid constant poking while they were looking for a good vein to insert a needle into.

An implanted port (simply referred to as a "port") is like an artificial vein. It makes it easier for healthcare professionals to access blood vessels for medications and tests.

The port has many uses. It provides access to:

- Give intravenous (IV) medication.

- Draw blood for tests.

- Give you chemotherapy continuously for several days.

  - Sometimes, chemotherapy must be given in a vein larger than the ones in a person's arms. The port allows the medication to be delivered into the bloodstream through a large vein near their heart.

The port, located near the front of my left shoulder does not show through the skin, though it can be felt by a light touch which makes it easily accessible for medical professionals. It is implanted through a short surgery procedure which does not require an overnight hospital stay.

It is expected to remain in my body for years as I continue to have regular blood checks looking for indications of additional cancer.

# Body healing before port surgery

Like the window between my radiation treatment and the first surgery, I was into another time period when it was important for my body to be ready to take the chemo but not have too much scar tissue forming from my initial surgery to interfere with the chemicals reaching all parts of my body. The timing was important to get any remaining cancerous lymph nodes before they had a chance to spread to vital organs.

The "window" they provided was around 4 – 6 weeks from my colon surgery until beginning IV chemo. It sounds pretty simple, but like other parts of my cancer treatment, it had some complications.

When I went to the surgeon on a follow-up visit from my hospital stay, she checked the stitching on my rectum and found the stitches were pulling away from some skin – in other words my stitches were acting like a zipper becoming undone and there was a lot of bleeding.

She repaired the stitching (zipped the zipper) but was not satisfied with the healing process. The radiation had changed some skin making it puffy and unable to hold stitches without coming apart again and it was unlikely to be healed enough to have a port installed and begin the IV treatment on time. So off I went to another specialized medical professional, a Doctor specializing in Wound Care and Hyperbaric treatment.

## Wound Doctor

There is apparently a field of medicine specializing in wound repair – helping wounds that don't want to heal such as my radiated skin.  I was sent to a person I refer to as a wound doctor to see if he could help my skin return to its original condition so it could connect properly to the stitches.

Due to the critical timing to begin my IV chemo treatment, the doctors involved suggested using a Hyperbaric Chamber.

Hyperbaric Oxygen Therapy:

Body tissues need an adequate supply of oxygen to function.  When tissue is injured, it requires even more oxygen to survive.

Hyperbaric oxygen therapy (sitting in a pressurized chamber) increases the amount of oxygen a person's blood can carry.  An increase in blood oxygen temporarily restores normal levels of blood gasses and tissue function to promote healing and fight infection.
(Source:  Mayo Clinic/Internet)

*In my case, the Hyperbaric Chamber did not happen.*  It was too soon after my radiation treatment to be covered by insurance – the Wound Doctor went for plan B.

## Wound Doctor – Plan B

Without the option of the Hyperbaric Chamber, the Wound Doctor decided to treat my radiated flesh with silver. The medical terminology is: topical antimicrobial dressing. The laymen's terminology (my interpretation) is that he put a dressing over my radiated skin that contained silver (yep! Just like silverware and jewelry).

Author's warning:

A silver dressing is special <u>sanitary dressing</u> like a gauze pad with silver imbedded in it – so don't try treating a wound by sticking a fork in your arm to speed healing.

Healing with silver is apparently controversial in the world of medical science, but those who believe in using silver dressings for a slow healing wound believe it helps clean wounds and manage potential infection so the skin can heal more rapidly than simply leaving the wound covered with more traditional dressings.

Controversial or not, it worked. It required a few weeks of visiting the Wound Doctor and having the silver dressing changed in the Doctor's office and by the home Visiting Nurse, but the skin healed in time to support the port surgery and IV Chemo process – and much to my delight, they were able to remove all of the stitches I'd been sitting on for weeks and a constant sharp pain left with the stitches.

Silver is a precious metal and an industrial commodity—but did you know that it also is a powerful healing agent? Silver has antimicrobial and antibacterial properties, and it has been used throughout the ages to cure infections and help heal wounds.

Now interest in silver is growing in the medical community because new studies have found that it can kill a wide range of bacteria and viruses, including the very dangerous *E-coli* and *Staphylococcus*.

> *Source:* Mark A. Stengler, ND, a naturopathic medical doctor and leading authority on the practice of alternative and integrated medicine.

If a person does some research on the healing qualities of silver they will find themselves reading about royal families of many years ago eating with silver to prevent a buildup of bacteria and disease in their mouth. It ties into the phrase about some people being born with "a silver spoon in their mouth."

# VERTIGO
## (Not the Alfred Hitchcock movie)

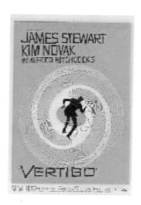

Vertigo – the medical variety
> "...a sensation of feeling off balance.  Dizzy spells that make a person feel like they are spinning or the world around them is spinning." (Source: WebMD)

Every time I felt like I was recovering and doing well, I seemed to find a new challenge in my life.  The next challenge I found was vertigo.

During my "rest period" while caring for my silvery wound and thinking about the upcoming port surgery, I woke up one morning and everything was normal – *then I sat up.*

> All of a sudden I felt like the room was spinning in one direction and I was spinning in another.  I held on to the bed and sat until the spinning stopped, then I tried to function with my regular morning routine.

For the rest of the morning, every time I would tilt my head the spinning would start again.  Eventually I fell in the kitchen and my head left a dent in our newly painted kitchen.

I did not hit anything else, only the wall, inches from a sharp cornered piece of furniture, but I missed it.

As the room stopped spinning my thought processes were focused on the money we had just paid to have the kitchen remodeled vs. repairing my head – and I was more concerned about the wall than I was my head. I figured all of the specialized Doctors I had met so far could fix my head, but finding a sheet rocker for a small dent in a wall is more of a challenge.

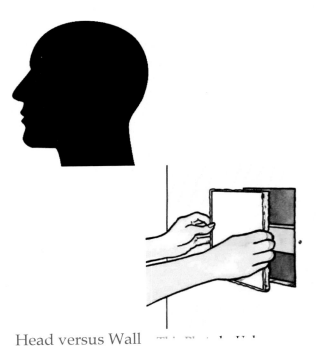

Head versus Wall

It was a Sunday when I hit my head, so there was not much point in trying to reach our Primary Care Physician. My head did not seem to be as damaged as the wall, so there was no need to go to an Emergency Room. Our next choice was a nearby Urgent Care facility – new adventure for us but we thought I should see a Doctor to find out why my world was spinning so much.

Like nearly all the other medical professionals we had met in recent months, the staff and Doctor at the Urgent Care facility were very efficient and very nice. There was only a short wait to see the Doctor.

After a few tests looking at my eyes and checking vital signs, the diagnosis was "vertigo." The cause is not necessarily known, but it will usually go away in a few days on its own. The spinning can be minimized with some prescription pills.

> Apparently vertigo is the result of a few crystals in the inner ear leaning sideways when they should be pointing straight up. They are very small (4 can be balanced on the point of a pin) but critical to helping the ear keep us in balance.

In addition to waiting for the crystals to right themselves, there is a controversial cure which is done by a Physical Therapist. They hold a patient's head rigid and give it a quick turning motion to jar and realign the crystals that have become slanted, or off balance.

The pills from the Urgent Care Doctor did not seem to do much for me and my world kept on spinning, so I made an appointment with our Primary Care Physician. She gave the same diagnosis, vertigo, and shared more information about treatment by a Physical Therapist.

Next, I went to a Physical Therapist. He did a few tests while watching my eyes, then did the head jerk treatment. My vertigo went away almost immediately, but my mental attitude toward falling had me shaken up and unsure of my own abilities.

> Nobody will share their opinions about how I got vertigo, but my though is that it probably related to being "suspended upside down" for several hours in surgery.

## MORE SURGERY – INSTALL PORT

Based upon trying for a 90% chance of getting all of the cancer when I agreed to Chemo IV treatments, I was actually agreeing to 8 "drip" sessions over 16 weeks.

The routine for each session was to have a blood draw every other Monday, then a 3 ½ hour session on Tuesday with a series of IV drips. I would go home with an external pump connected to my port into a tube ending near my heart, then return on Thursday to remove the pump and have another 1 hour IV drip. I would take the next week of for recovery and return in two weeks to repeat the drip series.

All of my IV drips were done through a port (access point) near my shoulder so they did not have to search for veins every time I went for treatment. So – in order to have a port available to the IV nurses, I needed more surgery to install the port.

## The port surgery

The surgery to install a port was accomplished in the same hospital area by the same surgeon. This time they were very aware of my earlier pneumonia so the Anesthesiologist explained I would be laying on my back with my head down and a breathing tube in my mouth. As usual, I said I was OK with whatever they did, I just did not want to see any of it.

Again, the conversation I remember with the Anesthesiologist was "I'm OK with." The next part of the conversation was "it's time to wake up."

I was moved into a recovery room with my wife by my side where I recovered quickly and was ready to go home by early afternoon. The recovery nurse arranged a wheel chair to get me to our truck, we both got in with my wife in the driver's seat, and the nurse left with a kind smile and wave.

My wife turned the ignition key -- nothing happened. Our battery (an almost new battery) did not have enough power to start the engine. Thank goodness for AAA. We called, they came to give us a jump start and we headed for home.

It was a nice sunny day, so while waiting for AAA in the hospital parking lot we just enjoyed the freedom of being outside, breathing fresh air, and being together. We knew AAA was coming, so no need to be concerned.

All of the hospital and medical visits up to this time had occurred in late Fall and Winter and she had been driving with the heater, windshield wipers, headlights, and music on nearly every day. Our home is a short drive from the hospital so it was not long enough to fully charge the battery.

We made it home safely, I managed to have some rest, then five days later I entered another entirely different world of cancer treatment – the IV lab.

# THE IV LAB

I'm not sure I have the name of the unit right, so I'll just refer to the area where patients go for their IV procedures as the IV Lab. It is a world in cancer treatment like no other place I had ever visited or experienced.

The room is very large with eight tilting chairs (can be used for sitting upright or laying back) around the walls, each one with a sliding privacy curtain around it. The curtains are generally open so each patient can look out the window to a very comforting landscape, as well as make eye contact with other patients. Each chair has a rolling IV pump stand next to it which is normally plugged into a wall socket but can be moved with an attached battery for restroom breaks, etc.

The center of the room has a large nursing station for the staff. It is surrounded by a counter which is low enough for every staff member to be able to watch patients in every chair.

When I went into the room, every chair with the exception of one (mine) had a patient in it with tubes connecting them to several dripping bags. I eventually began referring to the other patients as my "drip mates" and got to recognize several of them over time.

## Project Management and Teamwork

While resting in my chair and reading a book, I was able to spend a lot of time watching the activity in the room. It was an outstanding example of Project Management and well coordinated staff Teamwork.

> **Project management** is the discipline of initiating, planning, executing, controlling, and closing the work of a team to achieve specific goals and meet specific success criteria. ... The primary challenge of **project management** is to achieve all of the **project** goals within the given constraints.

> **Teamwork** in health is **defined** as two or more people who interact interdependently with a common purpose, working toward measurable goals that benefit from leadership that maintains stability while encouraging honest discussion and problem solving.

I have to be careful writing this section because I do not want it to sound like a college lecture. With a business career that included several years as a Project Manager and later as a college Professor who taught Project Management, it would be difficult for me to not discuss the outstanding coordination and team effort I witnessed every day in the IV Lab. It reminded me of a quote from Pete Carroll, Coach of the Seattle Seahawks in his book *Win Forever – Live, work, and play like a champion:*

> "...as a team we couldn't have been closer...we all grew up and learned together and our effort was the culmination of the ideas we had conceived and worked so hard to build." (Page 166)

The IV Lab at the St. Anthony Hospital Cancer Center is an outstanding example of both Project Management and Teamwork.

> The lab itself is very clean and designed with all of the supplies the Nurses and staff need to do their work located for convenient access with inventory constantly being checked and restocked throughout the day.

> Every person working in the IV Lab has a work station with the equipment and technology (computer system) they need to do their task.
> Nurses and staff work stations are arranged so people with similar responsibilities are near each other so they converse and share ideas when necessary.

> Everyone working in the IV Lab is constantly watching patients and paying attention to other staff members. Every one of them are quick to back up any other staff member if a patient needs help or has a drip bag alarm going.

They are all very friendly and go out of their way to make each patient feel well cared for – and they all share a comfortable sense of humor which helps develop a lot of smiles in an otherwise high stress environment.

## Starting the IV procedure – blood draw

The day before receiving the actual IV drip, I would always go to the lab and have a blood draw. The results of the draw were provided to the Oncologist and hospital Pharmacist to review, adjust, and prepare the drip bag to be used the next day.

## The IV drip

The day after the blood draw was the actual start of each IV procedure. I found the actual IV procedure very relaxing. Except for a very quick needle prick at the beginning, I never felt anything in the entire process.

It was so relaxing it could actually be a bit boring without a book, some writing material, or some other small form of entertainment to help pass the time. My biggest concern was trying to keep from falling asleep and bothering people with my snoring (it relates to a very definite side effect which is constantly being tired – lot of short naps helps).

> If you are a patient and you bring something to do while you are in a chair receiving an IV drip, remember your work space is limited. You will have a small tray on the arm of the chair, but it is about the size of an airline meal tray.

When I was in my chair, the Nurse inserted a needle into my port (people without a port received their Chemo IV in their vein) and connected tubes to several hanging bags. They set a timer on each bag – and that was that – I sat and read a book while the bags dripped.

When the bags were empty, the nurse returned and, in my case (it is different for each patient) they attached a new bag and a small external pump to my port. The bag and pump were placed in a fanny pack which I wore home and kept attached for two days.

After two days, I returned to the lab and had the external bag and pump removed. They connected another bag which dripped for about one hour. Then – I was finished and went home to enjoy a week without any medical procedures.

This routine went on every two weeks for 8 sessions (16 weeks) and in the process several things became common in the IV Lab that I think are worth sharing:

- Every visit to the IV Lab has a carefully coordinated schedule so, like with all of my other medical procedures, I never had to wait more than 10 minutes to be escorted to my assigned chair.

- Nurses tend to wear comfortable, but fun shoes. A lot of their shoes are bright colors and made me think of the phrase "happy feet".

- The Nurses and staff were constantly moving – though they had some time to have private conversations, they were absolutely dedicated to helping patients feel watched and cared for.

- The entire room enjoyed the therapy dog every time he would come to visit. Even patients who appeared to be suffering a bit managed a smile when the dog went to see them.

- Sometimes visitors or people waiting to give a ride to patients brought treats (e.g. cupcakes, etc.) and when they did, they brought enough for everyone – staff and patients included.

- There was a feeling throughout the lab that showed everyone knew some tough cancer battles were going on, but we were all in it together and did all we could to keep everyone's spirits up.

- They had baskets full of snack food (crackers, chips, etc.) available for anyone to take and munch on while they are in their IV chairs. It was always interesting to watch people select their particular small bag of chips, cookies, etc. Most were very selective, while a few just reached in the basket and grabbed what was on top.

## Side Effects

### Tired

Other than being tired most of the time, I have not suffered what I would call major side effects from the Chemo pills or IV drips. I believe some of my tiredness is related to waking up several times a night worrying about my Colostomy bag working properly. As time goes by and I am getting more and more comfortable (but still not liking) the bag, I do find myself sleeping for longer stretches.

### Hair

I have not lost any hair (other than the genetic thing they refer to as "male pattern baldness") as a result of my cancer battle. My hair has stopped growing, but it is not falling out.

### Diet

I'm still adjusting to what is alright to eat and what is not necessarily good to eat. This is covered in more detail in the Dietician section. I have not had any lack of appetite.

## Cold

During our initial orientation at the beginning of the cancer battle, we were told I'd be sensitive to cold – I was, but we did not understand each other. I thought they were referring to external cold so in my mind I said to myself "big deal, it won't bother me." I have spent nights sleeping in igloos and snow caves without the cold bothering me, so I was not concerned about a little chill.

Warning!!! They were not referring to external cold. They were talking about internal – like inside my mouth. The first time I drank a glass of water from inside the refrigerator (so it was cold) my mouth REALLY reacted. I did not know there were so many sensitive places inside a mouth. I learned and it is alright now – I just let water, tea, etc. sit out and get to room temperature begore I drink it.

## Dizzy

My head has what I'd refer to as a permanent dizziness, or buzz going and it has been with me since the cancer treatments began with the pills taken along with my doses of radiation. It is not enough to stop me from functioning, but I am a bit careful.

There are some things I won't do with my fuzzy head, for example:

I mentioned early in this writing that I volunteer to help inmates at the local women's Correctional Center develop business plans to help them when they are released. As long as I have a "fuzzy head" I will not go near the Correctional Center. It is too important to be clear headed when I am working one-on-one with inmates.

While I am referring to the women inmates, I should point out that they have been very strong supporters in my cancer battle. I receive a lot of notes and prayers from them wishing me good luck as I continue the fight. They are amazing ladies. When I think about their current lifestyle and lack of freedom – they make my cancer battle seem pretty minor compared to what they have to live with each day for several years.

**Falling**

I found myself pretty unsteady on my feet and managed to fall a couple of times while walking across the lawn and in shopping mall parking lots.

(I felt foolish on the ground in a Wall Mart parking lot, trying to look casual, but that is a story for another time).

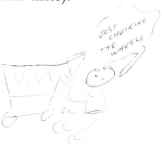

I believe the unsteadiness was in a lot of ways, the result of a fuzzy head and being tired most of the time – or just carelessness on my part.

I fell often enough (this was not spinning Vertigo – this was just tripping over my own feet) to visit our Primary Care Physician.

After some discussion about my years of climbing mountains, I told her I would like to be able to just walk comfortably on a groomed trail in a park setting. She gave me a prescription to have a Physical Therapist (PT) help me become more steady on my feet. I'll start with the PT effort after I have been off the Chemo IV for a few weeks and feel "almost" normal.

### Finger nails

Odd in my opinion, but while everything else in my body seemed to be slowing down or changing (skin getting dry and tight, hair stopped growing, etc.) my finger nails (not toe nails) began growing much faster than before, starting with the oral Chemo pills during my radiation treatment but they were thinner than normal and easy to break.

### Stomach pain and diarrhea

After a few weeks of the IV drips, I began to experience extreme pain near my stomach. It would start with pain near my stomach and expand to my lower back on both sides. I tried Tylenol and Ibuprofen – not together. They did not seem to help. I had difficulty standing or sitting. Eventually I learned the only relief I could find was to lay on my back.

Not long after the pain let up, I got into bouts of diarrhea that lasted about 24 hours. I mentioned it to the Oncologist during my regularly scheduled visit with him after a few weeks of suffering. He told me the best treatment is lying flat on my back and letting the body relax.

This is another example of where I did not listen to my own advice – I should have contacted the Cancer Navigator and asked who to go to for help. I didn't contact her and suffered a great deal for several weeks as a result.

They tell me the side effects will go away over time – by "time" they tell me it can vary – weeks, months, or in the case of some of the radiation pain – years.

# DIETICIAN

As I was reaching the end of my Chemo by IV, I was developing a lot of questions about "what happens next?" "What do I need to do keep my Colostomy bag working well throughout the rest of my life?" "Etc.?"

So, finally listening to my own advice – off I went to the Cancer Navigator for help – and once again she came through with the right direction at the right time.

She connected me with an Oncology Dietician – good move and highly recommended for any cancer patient.

The Dietician spent a lot of time with me and my wife explaining how the Colostomy world worked, what was good to eat, how to eat (smaller pieces, etc.), and what to avoid. She was very realistic in her advice and shared diet/nutrition ideas that will allow us to enjoy every meal, while being careful not to overdo it with some food groups in a single setting.

I learned a lot from the Dietician – and she left a welcome mat out for me to return anytime to share concerns and learn more about healthy eating.

# WHAT IS NEXT?

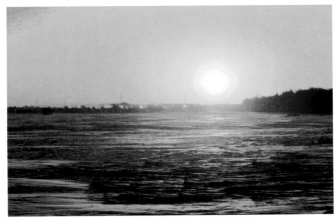

It is time to begin letting go of the past and begin dreaming about the future!

### End of treatment Oncologist visit

When I reached my last scheduled IV it was time for a visit with the Doctor I thought of as my primary Oncologist to discuss the status of my cancer battle and help me understand how the treatments would be followed up.

I have learned from past experience it helps a Doctor when I provide them (through their nurse) a typed set of questions and concerns I want to discuss in advance of our meeting, even if it is only a few minutes before we are together. It gets our conversation off to a good start – and provides a checklist to be sure all of the concerns were covered before our conversation ends.

My list for the post IV procedure phase was:

How long will it take for the chemicals to leave my body?

How/when will we know of the Chemo Infusion worked?

What is the next step (follow-up schedule and procedure?

How long should I keep the Port in?

What kind of pain pills are recommended (e.g. Tylenol, Ibuprofen)?

Which Dr. do I go to now?
Oncologist, Surgeon, Primary Care Doctor?

The discussion with the Oncologist went well and he said I am <u>now considered a Cancer Survivor</u>

Definition: Cancer Survivor

"One who remains and continues to function during and after overcoming a serious or life-threatening disease. In cancer, a person is considered to be a *survivor* from the time of diagnosis until the time of death."

Not quite the definition I would like – I'd rather hear "cancer free," but I guess I'll take it as it comes and try to delay the "death" part for a few more years.

It is time to focus on the future and try to get back to the lifestyle and mental attitude that was in place nearly a year ago when I was told I had cancer. It will take time, but I'll work on it. I'm not sure I even remember what our "normal routine" was or will become.

## Acknowledgements

This booklet could not have been written and produced without the help of Jenna Berry, RN, MN, OCN, the Cancer Nurse Navigator at St. Anthony Hospital in Gig Harbor, Washington. Jenna was a vital resource as I wound my way through the somewhat confusing world of Cancer Treatment.

## Sources of material

Photographs and sketches in this booklet were created by the author or were taken with the author's camera.

## About the author

Richard (Dick) Larkin, a cancer survivor, lives with his wife of 50+ years in Port Orchard, Washington where they share their home with a friendly cat and they share their garden with neighborhood deer.

# GOOD LUCK ON YOUR OWN JOURNEY ENJOY EACH DAY, WHEREVER IT MAY LEAD

Keep a sense of humor – it does not hurt to smile and many times it helps people around you feel a little better.

Made in the USA
San Bernardino, CA
25 April 2018